BRILLIANCE BEAM PUBLISHING

Radiant Glow Skincare Secrets

Discover Natural Secrets For A Luminous Complexion that Boost Complexion And Reveals Your Best Self

First edition

This book was professionally typeset on Reedsy.
Find out more at reedsy.com

Contents

1

Introduction

In the realm of skincare, two souls intertwine their journeys: Valentine Nwachukwu and his beloved wife, Dessie. Together, they embark on a radiant odyssey, delving into the art of nurturing their skin and embracing a lifestyle of vitality. Their shared passion for healthy living serves as the cornerstone of their bond, igniting a desire to impart their wisdom to others. With hearts intertwined and spirits ablaze, they set forth to pen a testament to their experiences—chronicling the secrets that have bestowed upon them luminous skin and unwavering confidence.

Welcome to our first published book **"Radiant Glow Skincare Secrets,"** your very own simple and easy treatments and guide for attaining vibrant, healthy skin using simple yet effective tips and techniques.

In this book, we will explore the importance of nutrition, hydration, and lifestyle choices in promoting radiant and healthy skin that makes you feel confident and beautiful.

2

Hydration - Drink Up for Glowing Skin

Water is not only crucial for maintaining overall health but also plays a pivotal role in ensuring the vitality of our skin. When our bodies are dehydrated, our skin can suffer, leading to dryness, lacklustre appearance, and increased susceptibility to wrinkles. However, by prioritizing hydration, we can significantly improve the health and appearance of our skin, helping it to look vibrant and feel its best. Here are simple straightforward strategies to boost your daily water intake.

Carry a reusable water bottle with you throughout the day to remind yourself to drink more water.

We usually flavor our water with slices of lemon, cucumber, or berries for a refreshing twist.

We always set reminders on our phone or watch to take water breaks regularly, whether we are at home or at work.

Eat water-rich foods like watermelon, cucumbers, and oranges to help stay hydrated.

By making hydration a priority, you will not only improve the health of your skin but also boost your overall well-being.

3

The Power of Nutrients - Fuel Your Skin

Vitamins and minerals play a crucial role in maintaining healthy skin. Here are key nutrients and their benefits for your skin:

Vitamin A: Supports skin cell turnover and helps regeneration, in keeping your skin looking fresh and youthful. Carrots, sweet potatoes, and spinach are rich in vitamin A.

Vitamin C: Helps to brighten and even out skin tone, while also supporting collagen production for firmness and elasticity. Sources include citrus fruits, strawberries, and bell peppers.

Vitamin D: Plays a role in skin repair and helps to maintain the skin's barrier function. You can get vitamin D from sunlight exposure as well as fortified foods like dairy products and fortified cereals.

Vitamin E: Acts as a powerful antioxidant, protecting the skin from damage caused by free radicals. Nuts, seeds, and leafy greens are excellent sources of vitamin E.

Zinc: Supports skin healing and helps to regulate oil production, making it beneficial for acne-prone skin. Oysters, beef, and lentils are reliable sources of zinc. Incorporating a variety of nutrient-rich foods into your diet will provide your skin with the essential building blocks it needs to stay healthy and radiant.

4

Omega-3 - The Skin's Best Friend

Omega-3 fatty acids are essential fats that play a crucial role in maintaining skin health. They help to keep the skin hydrated, reduce inflammation, and support overall skin function. Here is how you can add more omega-3s to your diet.

Fatty fish like salmon, mackerel, and sardines stand out as exemplary sources of omega-3 fatty acids, essential for overall health and particularly beneficial for skin nourishment. Incorporating these fish into your diet provides a direct and potent source of omega-3, supporting skin hydration and radiance from within.

In addition to fatty fish, **Flax seeds and Chia Seeds** offer a plant-based alternative rich in alpha-linolenic acid (ALA), another type of omega-3 fatty acid. These seeds provide a convenient way to boost your omega-3 intake, adding nutritional depth to your meals and supporting skin health.

Walnuts also serve as a delicious and accessible source of omega-3. By consistently including walnuts in your diet, you can effortlessly enhance your omega-3 intake, further promoting skin hydration and radiance.

For those who may struggle to obtain enough omega-3 through dietary sources alone, **Supplements** like fish oil or algae oil can provide a convenient solution. Incorporating these supplements into your routine ensures that you meet your omega-3 needs, supporting both your overall health and the appearance of your skin.

By incorporating these omega-3 rich foods and supplements into our diet, we prioritize the holistic well-being of our bodies, resulting in a hydrated, nourished, and radiant complexion that reflects our commitment to skin health and vitality.

5

Probiotics - Nourish Your Gut, Nourish Your Skin

Embark on a captivating exploration into the intricate relationship between gut health and the luminous glow of our skin! Within the vast landscape of our gut microbiome, an ecosystem teeming with diverse microbial life, lies the secret to unlocking radiant skin. Probiotics, the superheroes of beneficial bacteria, stand as stalwart guardians of gut harmony, orchestrating a symphony of wellness within our bodies. Through the judicious inclusion of probiotic-rich foods in our diet, we fortify our inner ecosystem with the essential nutrients required for optimal gut health. This strategic nourishment forms the bedrock upon which our skin's vitality and luminosity thrive, emanating an unmistakable aura of clarity and radiance. Journey with us as we uncover the treasure trove of probiotic delights that we seamlessly integrate into our daily culinary repertoire, illuminating the path to skin brilliance from deep within.

Yogurt: Look for varieties that contain live and active cultures for maximum probiotic benefit.

Kefir: This fermented dairy drink rich in probiotics can be enjoyed on its own or mixed into smoothies.

Sauerkraut: Fermented vegetables like sauerkraut are rich in probiotics and can be a tasty addition to salads and sandwiches.

Kimchi: A fundamental component of Korean cuisine, kimchi is a zesty fermented cabbage dish abundant in probiotics.

Do not forget that incorporating probiotic-rich foods into your diet, you can also consider taking a probiotic supplement to support gut health and promote clear and glowing skin. We also add a balanced diet that is rich in whole foods in our food, which is very essential for supporting healthy, radiant skin. Below are tips for making healthier food choices.

Focus on Fruits and Vegetables: Strive to create a colorful masterpiece on your plate by dedicating half of it to an array of vibrant fruits and vegetables at every mealtime. These nutrient-packed foods are bursting with vitamins, minerals, and antioxidants, serving as potent nourishment for your skin from within. Embrace this wholesome dietary habit as part of your evening ritual, ensuring that each night before you retire to bed, you indulge in nature's bounty to promote skin health and radiance from the inside out.

Choose Whole Grains: When making dietary choices, consider incorporating whole grains like brown rice, quinoa, and oats into your meals. These grains are not only delicious but also packed with essential nutrients and fiber that contribute to overall well-being. By opting for whole grains over refined options, you are providing your body with a sustained source of energy and promoting digestive health. Additionally, the abundance of vitamins, minerals, and antioxidants found in these grains supports various bodily functions, including immune system function and heart health. Embrace the versatility of whole grains in your diet to nourish your body from within and support a healthier, more vibrant lifestyle.

Include Lean Protein: Protein serves as an essential element in the complex mechanism of skin repair and rejuvenation, acting as the fundamental building blocks for the renewal and maintenance of cellular structures and tissues. When you prioritize lean sources of protein in your diet, like tender chicken, flavorful fish, versatile tofu, and hearty beans, you are not just nourishing your body with vital nutrients, but you are also making a conscious choice to minimize unnecessary fats. By incorporating these wholesome protein options into your meals, you are not only supplying your body with crucial amino acids necessary for various physiological processes but also providing it with the foundational support required for optimal skin health and revitalization. It is about more than just satisfying your hunger; it's about empowering your body to thrive and ensuring that your skin radiates with vitality and resilience.

Reduction of Processed Foods: Processed foods like sugary snacks, fast food, and packaged meals can be high in unhealthy fats, sugars, and additives that can contribute to skin problems like acne, inflammation, and excess calories which your body does not need. By making slight changes to your diet and focusing on whole, nutrient-dense foods. you can fuel your skin from within and promote a healthy, radiant complexion.

6

Aging Gracefully - Tips for Youthful Skin

As we grow older, our skin loses collagen and starts sagging and wearing out. While we cannot stop the aging process entirely, there are steps we can take to help keep our skin looking youthful for longer. There are secrets that have contributed to our youthful and radiant appearance. I will be revealing those tips to you shortly.

Protect Your Skin from the Sun: Sun exposure is a major contributor to premature aging, so it is essential to protect your skin from the sun's harmful UV rays. Wear sunscreen with SPF 30 or higher every day, seek shade during peak sun hours, and wear protective clothing like hats and sunglasses.

Stay Hydrated: Skin lacking hydration may manifest as dry, lack luster, and susceptible to wrinkles. Ensure you stay adequately hydrated throughout the day by drinking enough water, as mentioned previously, to maintain your skin's moisture from within.

Ensure Ample Sleep: Inadequate sleep can result in dark circles, puffiness, and other telltale signs of fatigue, prematurely aging your appearance. Strive for 7-9 hours of restorative sleep each night to support your skin's natural repair and rejuvenation processes.

Manage Stress: Chronic stress can take a toll on your skin, leading to breakouts, inflammation, and other skin problems. Find healthy ways to manage stress, such as exercise, meditation, or spending time with loved ones

Eat a Balanced Diet: Revitalize Your Skin: Embrace a Diet Bursting with Colorful Fruits, Fresh Vegetables, Lean Proteins, and Nourishing Fats! Fuel your skin with the vital nutrients it craves for a youthful and vibrant glow.

Exercise often: Unlock Your Radiance: Discover the Power of Exercise! Engage in this invigorating routine 3 - 4 times weekly to sustain your glow and vitality. Not only does exercise fortify the heart and enhance circulation, warding off risks of heart disease and stroke, but it also cultivates a resilient mind. Join the movement towards a healthier you!

7

Skin-Saving Habits - Avoiding Common Culprits

Discover the secrets to maintaining radiant, youthful skin by steering clear of certain undesirable habits. Avoiding these pitfalls has been crucial in our journey towards vibrant skin health, shielding against damage and premature aging. Stay tuned as we reveal these skin-saving tips below!

Avoid Smoking: Smoking can damage collagen and elastin fibers in the skin, leading to premature wrinkles and sagging. If you smoke, consider quitting to protect your skin's health.

Limit Alcohol Consumption: Excessive alcohol consumption can dehydrate the skin and lead to inflammation, redness, and other skin problems. Limit your alcohol intake to promote healthier, clearer skin.

Protect Your Skin from Pollution: Environmental pollutants like smog, smoke, and particulate matter can wreak havoc on your skin, leading to premature aging and other skin problems. Wear sunscreen and protective clothing when outdoors and consider using skincare products that contain antioxidants to help protect your skin from environmental damage.

Be Gentle with Your Skin: Harsh skincare products, hot water, and rough scrubbing can damage the skin's natural barrier and lead to irritation, dryness, and other issues. Use gentle, fragrance-free products and avoid over-exfoliating or scrubbing your skin too hard.

Practice Good Skincare Habits: Follow a simple skincare routine that includes cleansing, moisturizing, and protecting your skin from the sun every day. Choose products that are suitable for your skin type and address your specific concerns, whether it is acne, dryness, or signs of aging. By avoiding these common skin-damaging habits and adopting healthier alternatives, you can help protect your skin's health and maintain a youthful, radiant complexion for years to come.

Radiant skin boasts a smooth texture, uniform tone, and youthful appearance, free from blemishes, dark spots, and signs of aging, emitting a luminous glow. Obtaining radiant skin entails a blend of effective skincare practices, mindful lifestyle choices, and environmental factors, as previously mentioned.

In the quest for radiant skin, addressing specific skin concerns is paramount in unlocking the full potential of one's complexion. By understanding the underlying causes of dullness, uneven tone, dryness, and sensitivity, individuals can tailor their skincare routines to target these issues effectively. Whether through revitalizing ingredients, advanced treatments, or holistic approaches to skincare, radiant skin is attainable for all, regardless of their unique skin. Concerns. With patience, consistency, and a commitment to self-care, individuals care embarks on a transformative journey towards luminous, glowing skin that radiates with health and vitality.

8

Skincare Routine

A consistent skincare routine is the foundation of radiant skin. It involves cleansing, exfoliating, moisturizing, and protecting the skin from sun damage. Here is a simple skincare routine to follow:

Cleansing: Start your day by washing your face with a gentle cleanser to remove dirt, oil, and impurities. Choose a cleanser that suits your skin type – whether it is oily, dry, or combination.

Exfoliating: Exfoliation helps remove dead skin cells, revealing fresh, radiant skin underneath. Use a mild exfoliate 2-3 times a week to unclog pores and improve skin texture, do not do it in excess.

Moisturizing: Hydration is key to radiant skin. Apply a moisturizer suited to your skin type to keep it nourished and supple. Look for ingredients like hyaluronic acid and glycerine for added hydration.

Clean After Outdoor Activities: After exposure to pollutants or sweat, cleanse your skin thoroughly to remove dirt and impurities that can clog pores and dull the complexion.

Use Protective Gear: In harsh weather conditions, such as cold winds or dry air, protect your skin by wearing scarves, hats, and gloves. This helps prevent moisture loss and irritation.

Invest in Skincare Products: We recommend you go for a perfect skincare product with protective ingredients like antioxidants (vitamin C, E) and barrier-repairing agents (ceramides, niacin amide) to shield your skin from environmental damage.

9

Understanding Specific Skin Concerns

It is essential to grasp the intricacies of various skin concerns. Dullness, for instance, stems from factors like dead skin cell buildup, environmental stressors, and inadequate skincare routines. Uneven skin tone, on the other hand, may result from hyperpigmentation, sun damage, or inflammation. Dryness often arises from a compromised skin barrier, leading to moisture loss and flakiness. Moreover, sensitive skin requires gentle yet effective solutions to alleviate redness, irritation, and discomfort.

Tailored Solutions for Radiant Skin:

- **Dullness:**

Com-batting dullness necessitates revitalizing skincare rituals designed to exfoliate, brighten, and nourish the skin. Incorporating chemical Com-batting like AHAs (Alpha Hydroxy Acids) and BHA (Beta Hydroxy Acids) helps slough off dead skin cells, revealing a smoother, more radiant complexion. Additionally, antioxidant-rich serums and moisturizers protect against environmental aggressors while promoting cell renewal.

Regular use of brightening agents like vitamin C and niacin amide can further enhance luminosity, leaving the skin glowing with vitality.

• Uneven Skin Tone:

Addressing uneven skin tone requires a multifaceted approach that targets pigmentation irregularities and restores balance to the complexion. Incorporating ingredients like hydroquinone, kojic acid, and licorice extract can help fade dark spots and hyper pigmentation, resulting in a more uniform appearance. Moreover, sunscreen is paramount in preventing further sun-induced damage and maintaining the efficacy of treatment. In-office procedures such as chemical peels and laser therapy offer advanced solutions for stubborn pigmentation concerns, yielding significant improvements in skin tone and texture.

• Dryness:

Replenishing moisture and fortifying the skin barrier are paramount in combating dryness and restoring radiance to parched complexions. Opting for hydrating cleansers and toners infused with humectants like hyaluronic acid helps retain moisture and prevent dehydration. Emollient-rich moisturizers and facial oils provide a protective barrier, sealing in hydration and soothing dry, flaky skin. Additionally, incorporating ceramides, fatty acids, and cholesterol in skincare formulations reinforces the skin barrier, enhancing resilience and suppleness over time.

• Sensitive Skin:

Sensitive skin requires gentle and efficacious solutions that soothe inflammation, strengthen the skin barrier, and minimize reactivity.

Choosing fragrance-free, hypoallergenic skincare products formulated with soothing ingredients like chamomile, aloe Vera, and colloidal oatmeal helps alleviate redness and irritation. Moreover, incorporating anti-inflammatory agents such as niacin amide and green tea extract calms sensitivity while providing antioxidant protection. Patch testing new products and avoiding harsh exfoliates and irritants are essential in managing sensitive skin without compromising its radiance.

Advanced Treatments for Specific Concerns:

In addition to targeted skincare routines, advanced treatments offer innovative solutions for stubborn skin concerns that may require professional intervention. Chemical peels, for instance, utilize exfoliating agents like glycol acid and salicylic acid to resurface the skin, revealing a smoother, more radiant complexion. Laser therapy, including intense pulsed light (IPL) and fractional lasers, targets pigmentation irregularities and stimulates collagen production, yielding dramatic improvements in tone and texture. Micro needling, on the other hand, promotes skin renewal by creating controlled micro-injuries, triggering the skin's natural healing response, and enhancing product absorption for optimal results.

The Importance of Consistency and Patience:

While targeted solutions can yield significant improvements in specific skin concerns, achieving radiant skin requires patience, consistency, and an integrated approach to skincare. Establishing a daily routine that incorporates cleansing, exfoliating, moisturizing, and sun protection is fundamental in maintaining skin health and vitality. Moreover, adopting healthy lifestyle habits such as staying hydrated, eating a balanced diet, and managing stress levels can further support radiant skin from within.

As a couple, we dedicate ourselves to nurturing excellent skin. This entails teamwork, communication, and a mutual dedication to placing skin health and self-care at the forefront. By establishing a steady skin-care regimen, prioritizing skin health through nutrition, implementing stress management methods, and selecting high-quality skincare items, you can commence a quest towards luminous and healthy skin. Keep in mind that caring for your skin is not just about appearance; it is also about feeling confident and at ease in your own skin.

In today's fast-paced world, stress, pollution, and hectic schedules can take a toll on our skin, leaving it dull, tired, and in need of rejuvenation. This is where regular spa treatments can play a significant role in pampering and revitalizing our skin. Spa treatments offer a range of therapeutic benefits that go beyond mere relaxation, providing our skin with the care and attention it deserves. In this comprehensive guide, we will explore the diverse benefits of regular spa treatments for skin health and overall well-being.

10

Understanding Spa Treatments

Before delving into the benefits, it is essential to understand what spa treatments entail. Spa treatments encompass a variety of therapies and procedures designed to promote relaxation, rejuvenation, and overall body wellness. These treatments often include massages, facials, body scrubs, wraps, and specialized skincare procedures performed by trained professionals in a serene and tranquil environment.

Stress Reduction and Relaxation:

One of the primary benefits of regular spa treatments is stress reduction and relaxation. Stress can wreak havoc on our skin, leading to inflammation, breakouts, and premature aging. Spa treatments offer a sanctuary from the stresses of daily life, allowing us to unwind, relax, and recharge both mentally and physically. Massage therapies, in particular, help release tension from the muscles, improve blood circulation, and promote a sense of calm and well-being, which reflects positively on our skin's health and appearance!

Deep Cleansing and Detoxification:

Regular visits to the spa for facials and body treatments are part of our routine, which include deep cleansing and detoxification, essential for maintaining healthy skin. Professional aestheticism utilize specialized products and techniques to eliminate impurities, unclog pores, and exfoliate dead skin cells, resulting in fresh, smooth, and radiant skin. Facial treatments may involve steam, extraction, and customized masks designed to target specific skin concerns such as acne, dehydration, or aging.

Stimulating Circulation and Cell Renewal:

Massage therapies and body treatments offered at spas stimulate circulation and promote cell renewal, which is vital for maintaining youthful and glowing skin. Improved blood flow delivers oxygen and nutrients to the skin cells, helping to repair damage, boost collagen production, and accelerate the skin's natural regeneration process. This results in improved skin texture, tone, and clarity, as well as a youthful radiance that comes from within.

11

Conclusion

As we conclude our journey through the intricacies of skin health, it is essential to reflect on the wealth of knowledge we have acquired. Throughout this book, we have delved deep into the science behind healthy skin, explored the crucial role of essential nutrients, hydration, skincare habits, and lifestyle factors in maintaining radiant skin. We have also examined the influence of environmental factors, discussed natural remedies, professional treatments, and strategies for aging gracefully.

Armed with this comprehensive understanding, you are now equipped with the tools and insights necessary to take charge of your skin health journey. From understanding your skin's structure to implementing effective skincare routines, you have gained invaluable knowledge to make informed decisions and navigate the myriad of options available in the realm of skincare.

As you embrace a holistic approach to skin health, remember that true beauty emanates from within. Nourish your skin with nutrient-rich foods, hydrate diligently, and prioritize self-care practices that promote overall well-being. By incorporating these principles into your daily life, you can cultivate healthy, radiant skin that not only looks good but also feels confident and empowered.

As you embark on this continued journey towards vibrant skin health, remember that your skin reflects your inner vitality and well-being. Embrace the knowledge you have gained, and let it empower you to make choices that prioritize your skin's health and radiance for years to come. With dedication, consistency, and an integrated approach, you can confidently navigate the ever-changing landscape of skincare and emerge with skin that glows with vitality and resilience.

12

Appendices and Resources

- Glossary: Find explanations for any unfamiliar terms or concepts mentioned throughout the book.
- FAQs: Get answers to commonly asked questions about skincare, nutrition, and lifestyle.
- Further Reading: Explore additional resources, books, and websites for more information on promoting healthy skin.
- Index: Easily locate specific topics or keywords discussed in the book.

13

Acknowledgments

Thank you to all the experts, researchers, and contributors whose knowledge and expertise helped make "**Radiant Glow**" possible. We truly value your commitment to advocating for healthy skin.

www.ingramcontent.com/pod-product-compliance
Lightning Source LLC
Chambersburg PA
CBHW070756260726
48660CB00007B/3142